Math Riddles For Smart Kids

Math Riddles Puzzles And Brain Teasers for Kids And Family Will Enjoy

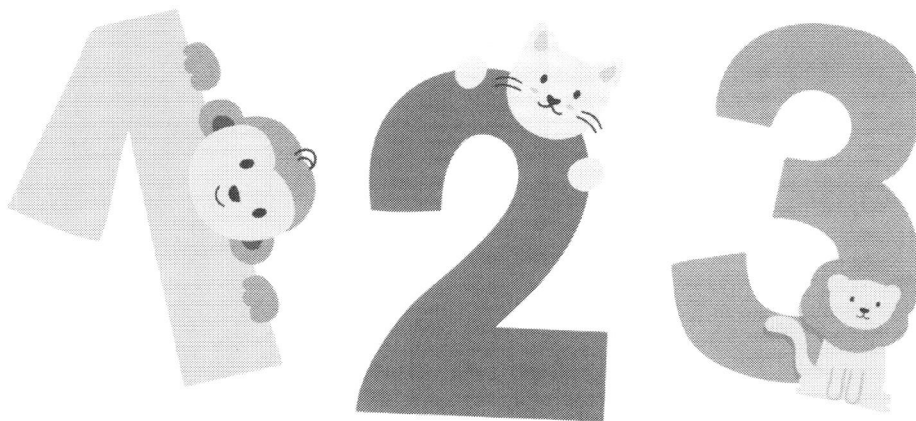

Henry Darwin

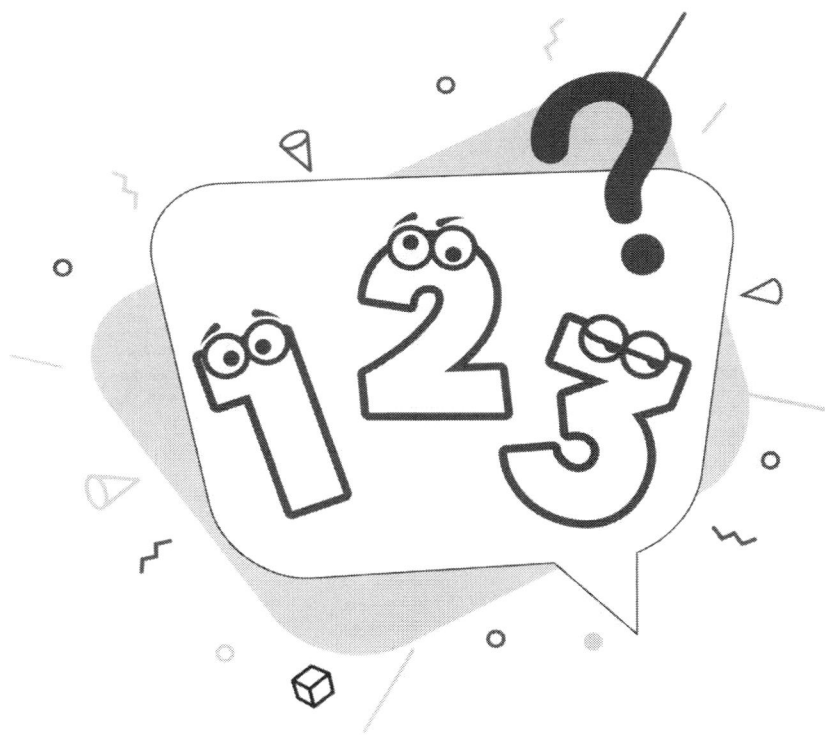

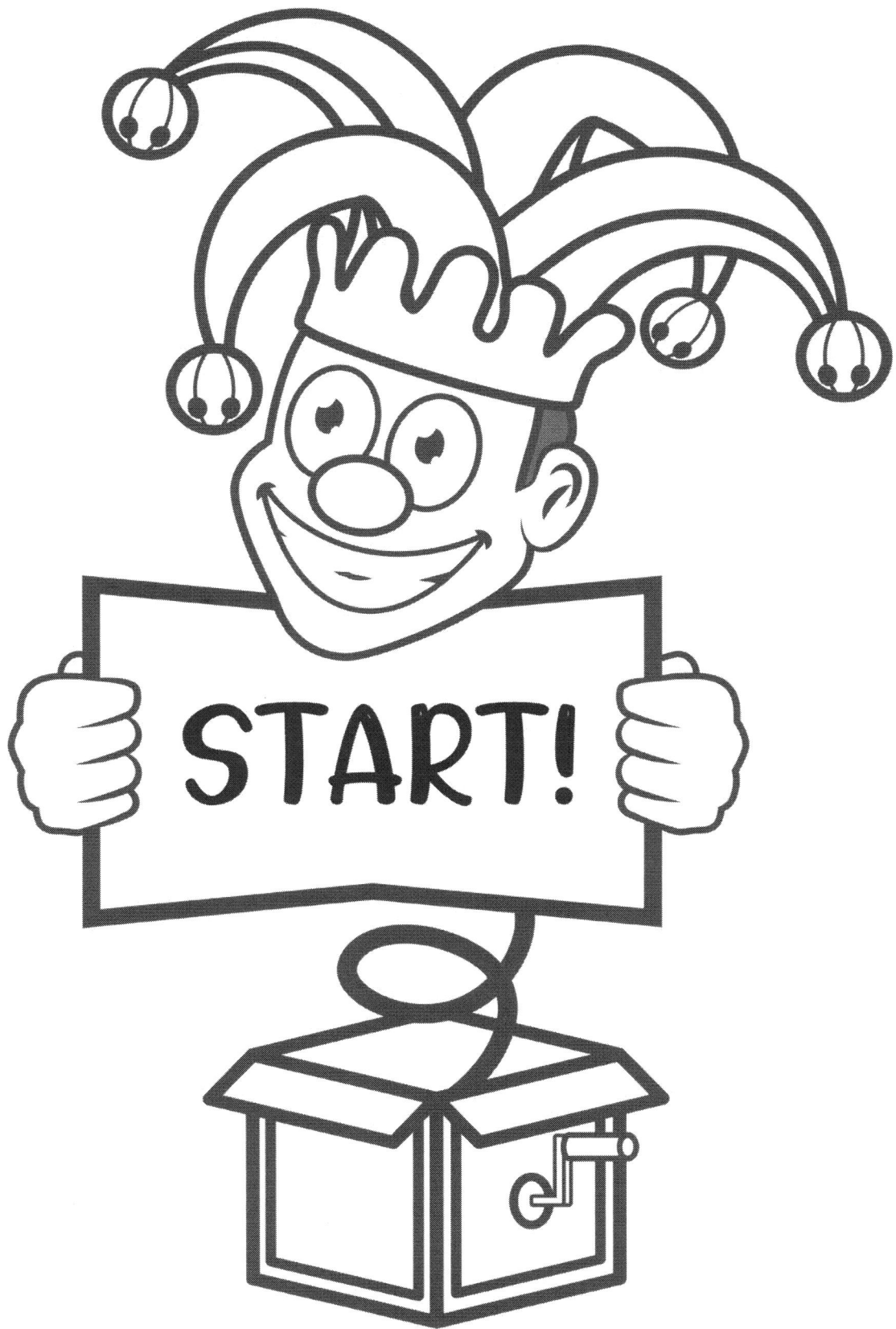

START!

Level 1

1. I am less than 10.
I am more than the number of sides on a triangle.
I am 2+2.
What number am I?

0 1 2 3 4 5 6 7 8 9 10

2. I am more than 2.
I am less than seven.
I am one more than the toes on one foot.
What number am I?

0 1 2 3 4 5 6 7 8 9 10

Level 1

3. I am between zero and 10.
I am more than two.
I am the number before 4.
What number am I?

0   1   2   ③   4   5   6   7   8   9   10

4. I am less than 20.
I am more than the number of days in a week.
I am 7+5.
What number am I?

1 2 3 4 5 6 7 8 9 10 11 ⑫ 13 14 15 16 17 18 19 20

Level 1

5. I am less than 10.
I am more than three.
I am the number of sides on two squares.
What number am I?

0   1   2   3   4   5   6   7   (8)   9   10

6. I am between 0 and 20.
I am more than 3+3.
I am the number of sides on two rectangles.
What number am I?

1 2 3 4 5 6 7 (8) 9 10 11 12 13 14 15 16 17 18 19 20

Level 1

7. I am between 2 and 10.
I am less than eight.
I am the number of sides on two triangles.
What number am I?

1 2 3 4 5 (6) 7 8 9 10 11 12 13 14 15 16 17 18 19 20

8. I am less than 15.
I am more than 6+3.
I am one less than thirteen.
What number am I?

1 2 3 4 5 6 7 8 9 10 11 (12) 13 14 15 16 17 18 19 20

Level 1

9. I am between 0 and 20.
I am more than the number of sides
on two rectangles.
I am 6+5.
What number am I?

1 2 3 4 5 6 7 8 9 10 (11) 12 13 14 15 16 17 18 19 20

10. I am between 0 and 15.
I am less than 10.
I am the number of days in one week.
What number am I?

1 2 3 4 5 6 (7) 8 9 10 11 12 13 14 15 16 17 18 19 20

Level 1

11. I am between 0 and 20.
I am more than the number of fingers on
two hands.
I am one less than 15.
What number am I?

1 2 3 4 5 6 7 8 9 10 11 12 13 14 15 16 17 18 19 20

12. I am between 0 and 15.
I am more than 4.
I am one less than 11.
What number am I?

1 2 3 4 5 6 7 8 9 10 11 12 13 14 15 16 17 18 19 20

Level 1

13. I am less than 15.
I am more than 6.
I am 10 – 2.
What number am I?

1 2 3 4 5 6 7 (8) 9 10 11 12 13 14 15 16 17 18 19 20

14. I am between 0 and 15.
I am less than nine.
I am two more than 4.
What number am I?

1 2 3 4 5 (6) 7 8 9 10 11 12 13 14 15 16 17 18 19 20

Level 1

15. I am between 0 and 20.
I am less than the number of fingers on two hands.
I am 2+5.
What number am I?

✓

1 2 3 4 5 6 7 8 9 10 11 12 13 14 15 16 17 18 19 20

16.   I am between 0 and 20.
I am more than 8.
I am 7+2.
What number am I?

✓

1 2 3 4 5 6 7 8 9 10 11 12 13 14 15 16 17 18 19 20

Level 1

17. I am between 0 and 20.
I am less than 15.
I am the number of sides on a triangle
and a square.
What number am I?

1 2 3 4 5 6 (7) 8 9 10 11 12 13 14 15 16 17 18 19 20

18. I am between 0 and 20.
I am more than the number of fingers on
one hand.
I am 6 + 4.
What number am I?

1 2 3 4 5 6 7 8 9 (10) 11 12 13 14 15 16 17 18 19 20

Level 1

19. I am between 2 and 20.
I am more than 12.
I am 13 + 1.
What number am I?

1 2 3 4 5 6 7 8 9 10 11 12 13 (14) 15 16 17 18 19 20

20. I am between 0 and 15.
I am less than 12.
I am 9 – 3.
What number am I?

1 2 3 4 5 (6) 7 8 9 10 11 12 13 14 15 16 17 18 19 20

Level 2

1. I am a number between 20 and 30. If you

count by fives, you will say my name. Who am I? 25 ✓

2. I am a number between 7 and 12. If you

count by threes, you will say my name. Who am I? ~~+6~~ 9 ✓

3. I am an even number. I am between 6 and 9. 8 ✓

Who am I?

4. I am a number less than 10. If you add me to 9 ✓

myself, you will find a number greater than 16. Who am I?

5. If you add me to 1, you will find

an odd number. I am less than 2. Who am I?

Level 2

16-10=6

6. 16 – 10 is less than I am. 16 – 8 is greater than I am.

Who am I?

7

7. If you subtract me from 14, you will find a

number greater than 11. I am an odd number. Who am I?

14 – 1 = 11 12, 13 14   7 13 ✓

8. I am an odd number. I am between 41 and 44.

Who am I?

43 ✓

9. If you add me to 50, you will find a number less than 70.

If you count by tens you will say my name. Who am I?

✓

60

7 + 7 = 14   7 + 9 = 15 16

10. 7 + 7 is less than I am. 7 + 9 is greater than I am.

Who am I?

15 ✓

Level 3

A grandmother, two mothers, and two daughters went to

a basketball game together and bought one ticket each.

How many tickets did they buy in total? 5

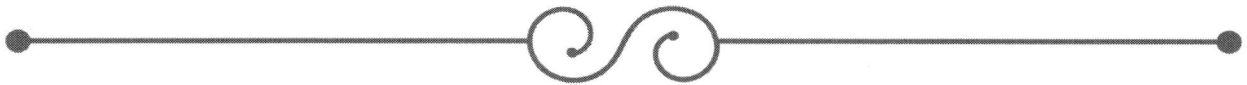

When Jackie was 6 years old, his little sister, Monica,

was half is age. If Jackie is 40 years old today,

how old is Monica? 40 and a half

Level 3

Add the number to the number itself and then multiply by 4. Again divide the number by 8 and you will get the same number once more. Which is that number?

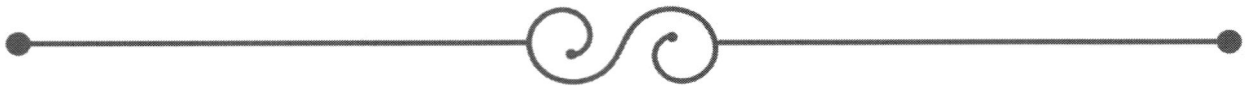

I add five to nine, and get two. The answer is correct, but how?

Level 3

Eggs are $0.12 a dozen. How many eggs can you get for a dollar?

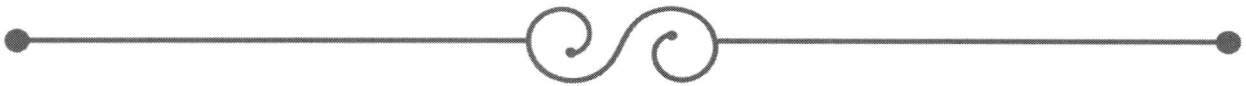

A man is twice as old as his little sister. He is also half as old as their dad. Over a period of 50 years, the age of the sister will become half of their dad's age. What is the age of the man now?

Level 3

The ages of a father and son add up to 66.

The father's age is the son's age reversed.

How old could they be?

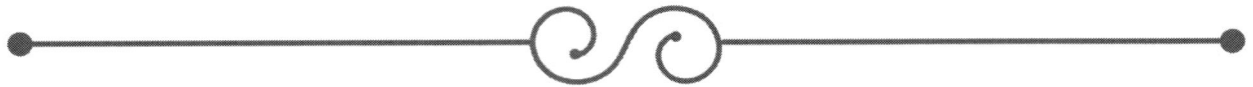

There are 100 pairs of bears in a zoo. Two pairs of babies are born for every dog. Unfortunately, 23 of the bears have not survived. How many bears would be left in total?

Level 3

Charlie has two kids. If the elder kid is a boy,

then what is the possibility that his other kid is also a boy?

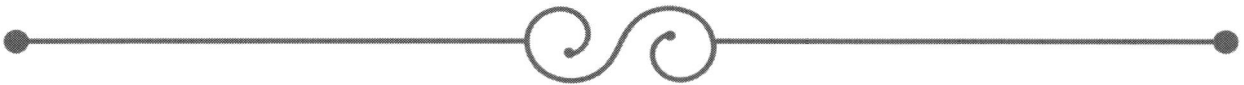

Velma has 7 daughters and each of them has a brother.

Can you figure out the total number of kids Velma have?

Level 3

A little boy goes shopping and purchases 12 potatoes.

On the way home, all but 9 get mushed and ruined.

How many potatoes are left in a good condition?

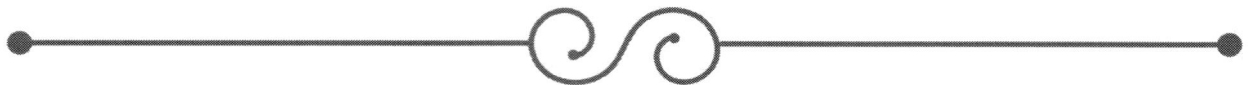

If you had five oranges and two apples in one hand and

two oranges and four apples in the other hand,

what would you have?

Level 4

1. Kevin turned 10 years old day before yesterday.

By next year he will become 13. How is this possible?

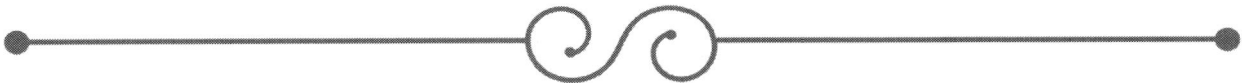

2. What is the following number?

18, 21, 24, 27, 30, 33, 36, _____

Level 4

3. What is the following number?

53, 51, 49, 47, 45, 43, _____

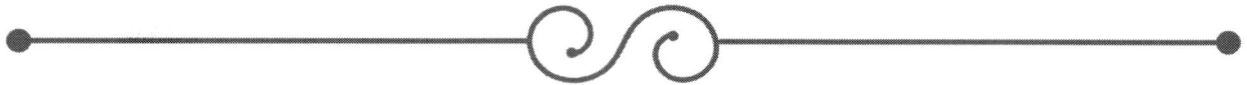

---

4. David had 6 siblings who were born all

born 2 years apart. The youngest is Lila who is

only 7 years old while David is the oldest.

What is David's age?

Level 4

5. Two fathers and two sons go fishing. Each of them catches one fish. So why do they bring home only three fish?

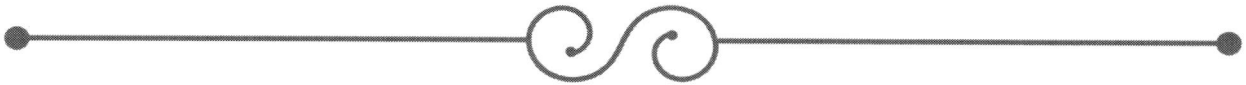

6. If Ella is the 50th fastest and slowest runner in her school, how many students are there in her school?

Level 4

7. Wolves and Lambs Puzzles: Six Wolves can catch just six lambs in six minutes. So how many wolves will they need to catch 60 lambs in sixty minutes?

Hint – the answer is not sixty.

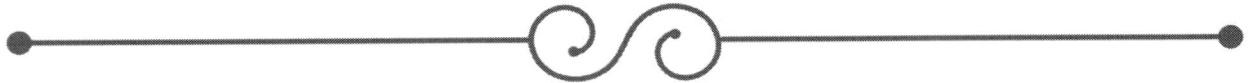

---

8. What do the numbers 88, 96 and 11 all have in common?

Level 4

9. There are 2 buckets, a 5 litre and a 3-litre bucket.

Fill the 5-litre bucket with 4 litres of water using just

these two buckets to measure.

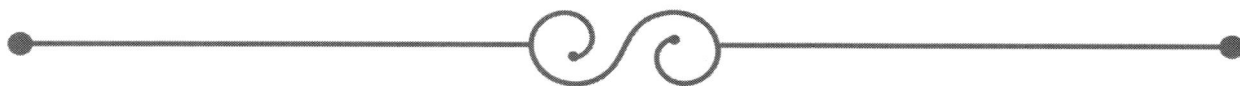

10. rabbit and carrots: Another word problem that is fun

for kids to solve. Assume there are, five rabbits and

each one takes 5 minutes to eat 5 carrots. How many

minutes would 4 rabbits take to eat 4 carrots?

Again, how many rabbits would eat 30 carrots

in 30 minutes?

Level 4

11. What weighs more – A kilo of apples or

a kilo of feathers?

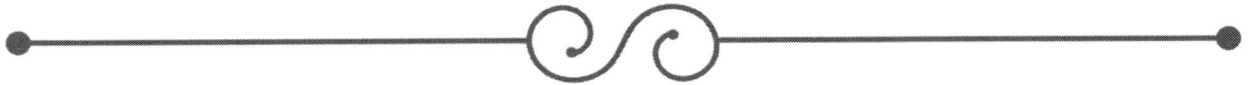

12. Using only addition, how can you add eight 8's to

get the number 1,000?

Level 4

13. The ages of a father and son add up to 66.

The age of the dad is the age of the son reversed.

How old could they be?

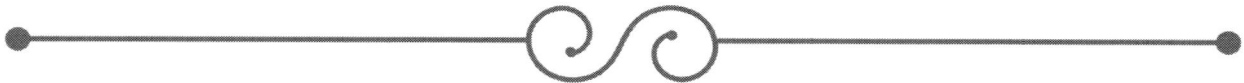

───────────────── ⟲⟳ ─────────────────

14. How many 9's are there between 1 and 100?

Level 5

1. When Grant was 8, his brother was half his age. Now, Grant is 14. How old is his brother?

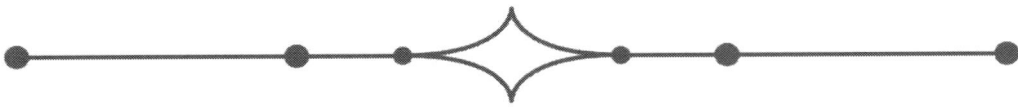

2. Two fathers and 2 sons spent the day fishing, but only caught 3 fish. This was enough for each of them to have one fish. How is this possible?

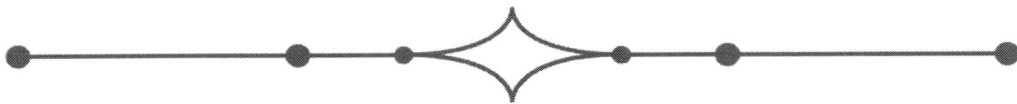

3. Leo was 11 the day before yesterday, and next year he'll turn 14. How is this possible?

Level 5

4. Isabella has 5 daughters. Each of these daughters has a brother. How many children does Isabella have?

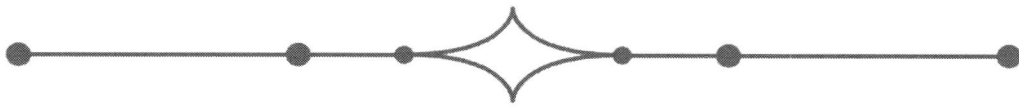

5. It's raining at midnight, but the forecast for tomorrow and the next day is clear. Will there be sunny weather in 48 hours?

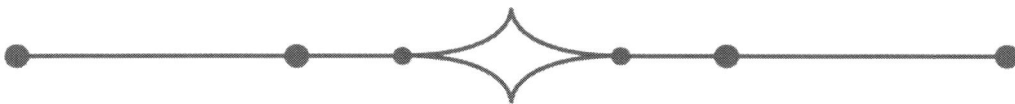

6. There are 3 apples in the basket and you take away 2. How many apples do you have now?

Level 5

7. What can you put between 7 and 8, to make

the result greater than 7, but less than 8?

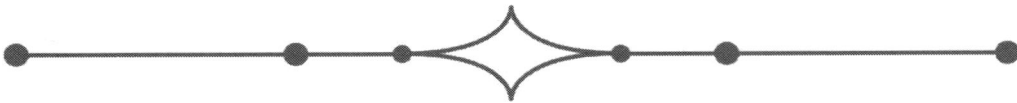

8. What 3 numbers give the same result when multiplied

and added together?

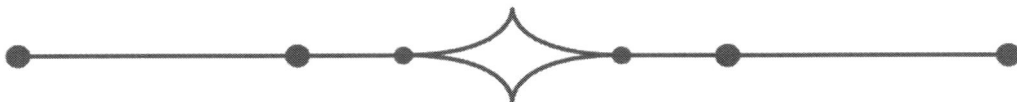

9. 81 x 9 = 801. What do you need to do to make

this equation true?

Level 6

1. Charlie used to live in a village that was next to the forest.

One day he crossed paths with a genie. The genie was in

a generous mood and granted Charlie one wish. Charlie, thinking

it was a joke, wished for a 100 grams of gold. The genie agreed

and behold! Charlie had a kilo of gold. Shocked and feeling upset

that he asked for so little, Charlie requested the genie if

he could ask for another wish. The genie agreed but only on one

condition. The genie would come back next month on any date

and Charlie would need to present him with gold rings.

However, the gold rings had to be the same weight as the date

on which he arrived. This means that if the genie came on

the 20th, he would need 20 grams of gold.

What did Charlie do next?

Level 6

2. How Many Cycles? This is another mathematical statement problem which can be solved using logic and arithmetic. Last weekend, Jack went to play in the park near his house. He rode the new bicycle gifted by his grandma on his birthday. After reaching the park, Jack saw that there were 14 tricycles and bicycles. If there were totally 38 wheels, how many tricycles were there in the park?

Level 6

3. Three brothers live in a farm. They agreed to buy new seeds: James and Thomas would go and Charlie stayed to protect fields. Thomas bought 75 sacks of wheat in the market whereas James bought 45 sacks. At home, they split the sacks equally. Charlie had paid 1400 dollars for the wheat. How much dollars did Thomas and James get of the sum, considering equal split of the sacks?

Level 6

4. In reply to an inquiry about the animals on his farm,

the farmer says: "I only ever keep sheep, pigs,

and horses. In fact, at the moment they are all sheep bar

three, all pigs bar four, and all horses bar five."

How many does he have of each animal?

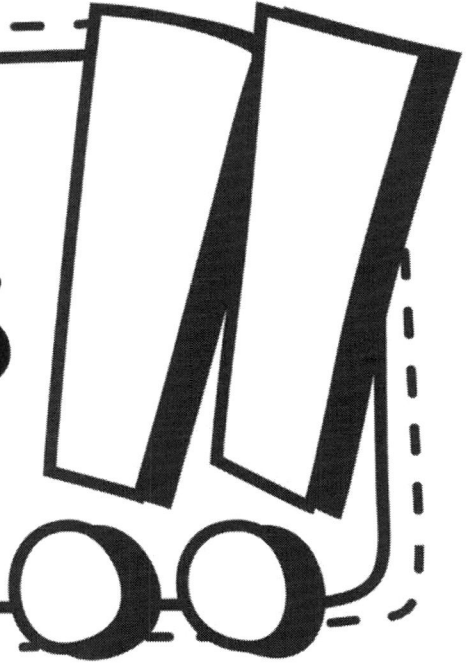

Bonus #1

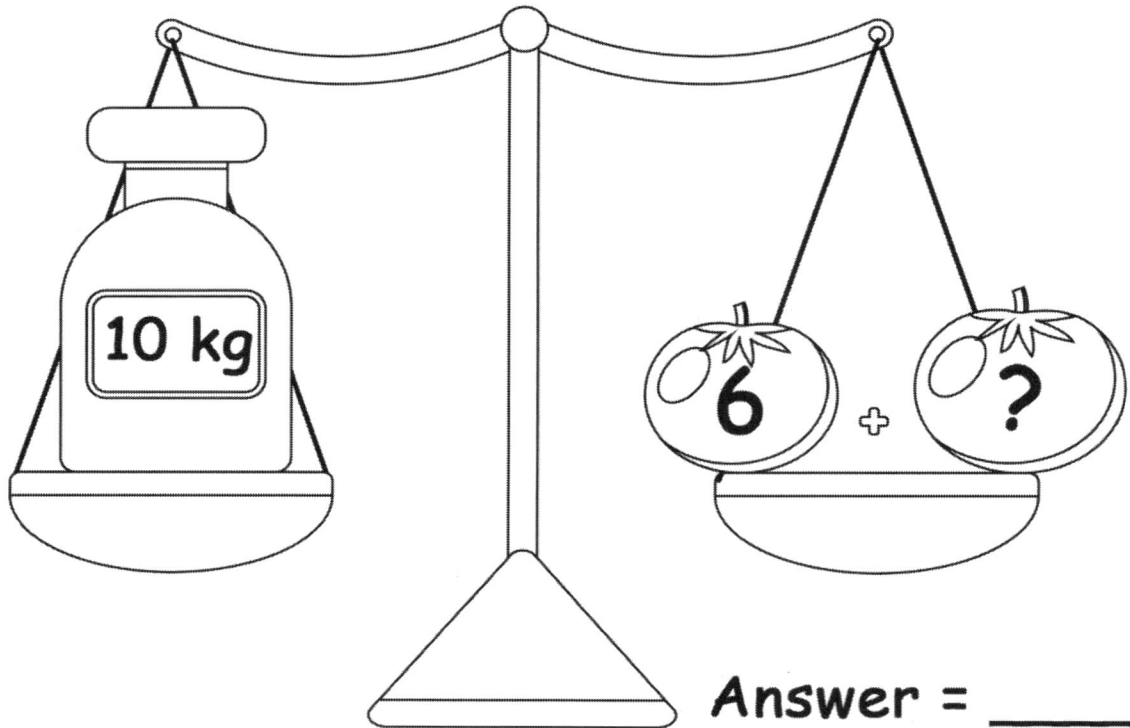

Answer = _____

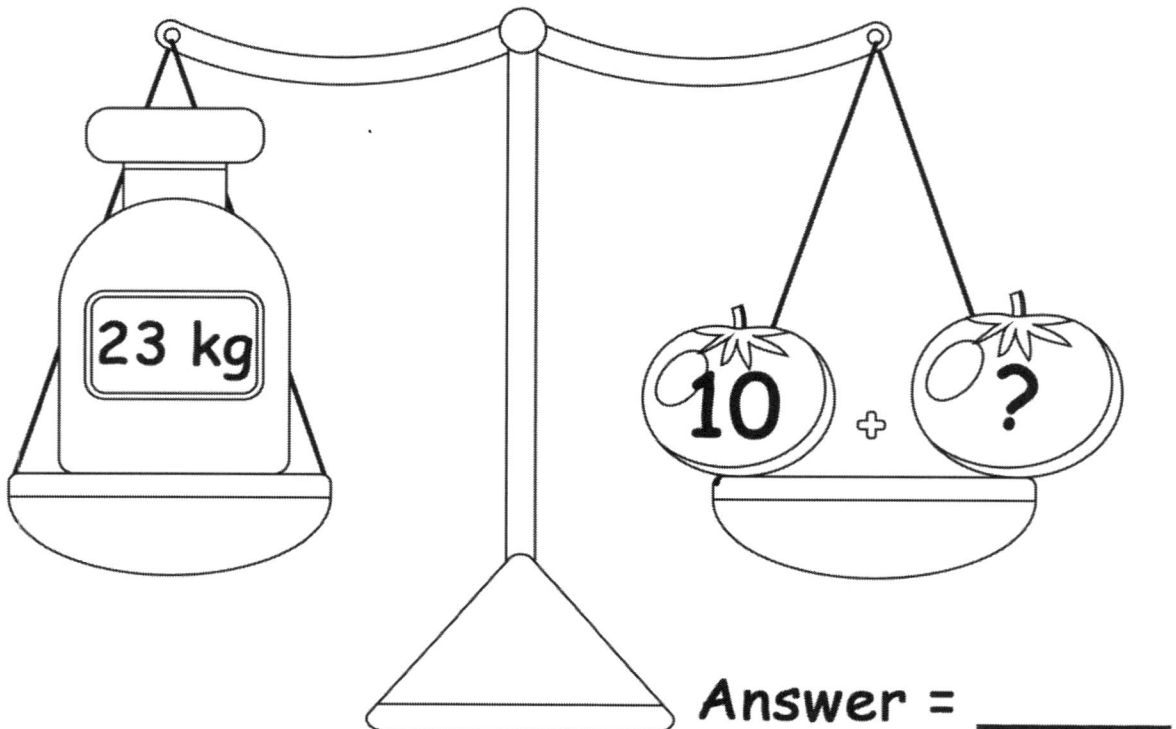

Answer = _____

Bonus #1

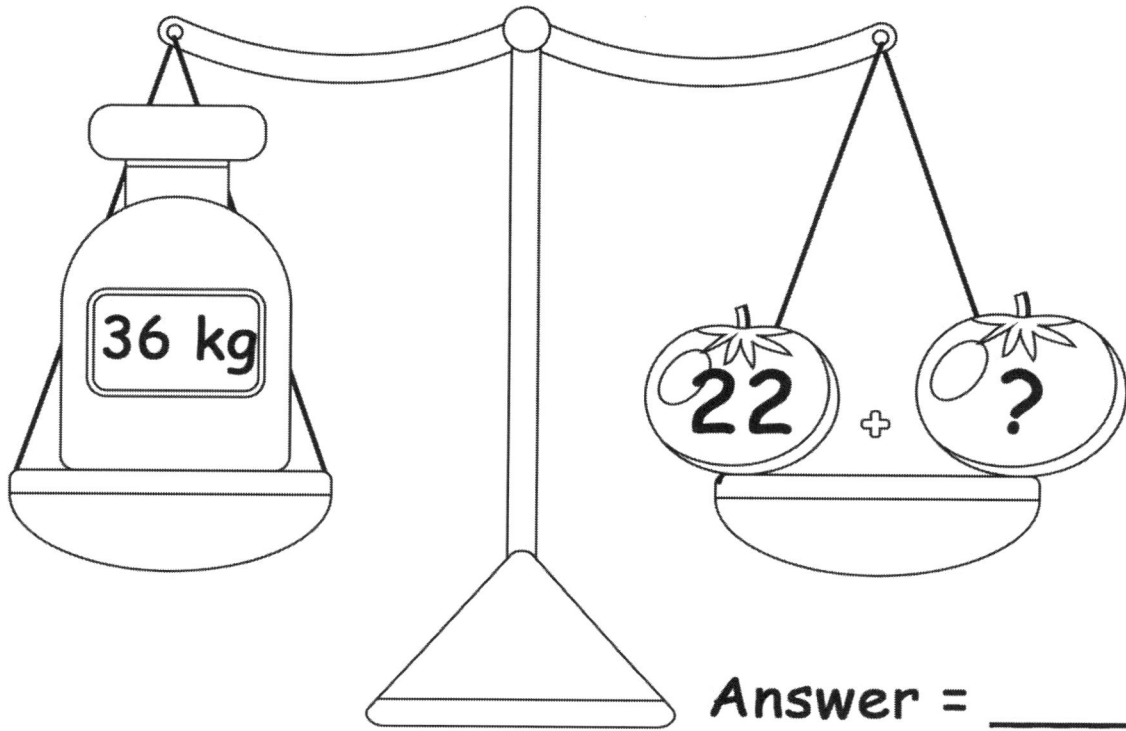

Answer = _____

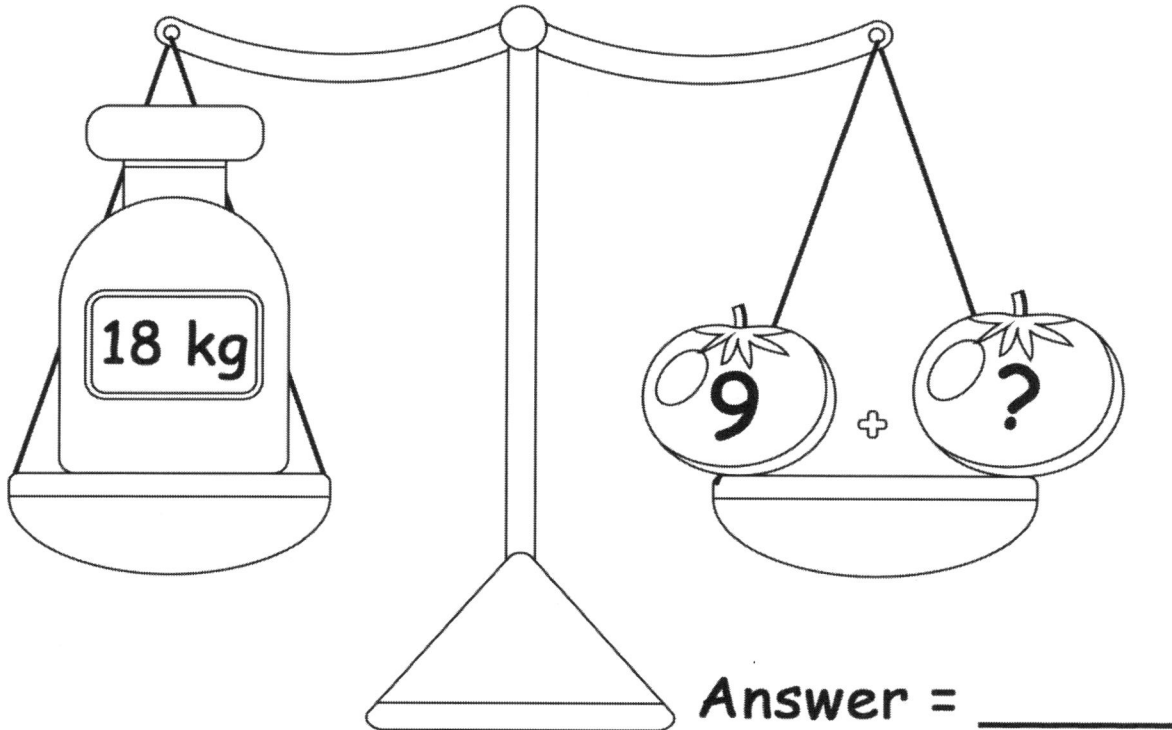

Answer = _____

Bonus #2

Replace mango with number 1, Replace grape with number 2,
Replace apple with number 3.
What is the answer to each question?

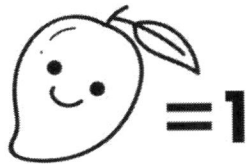

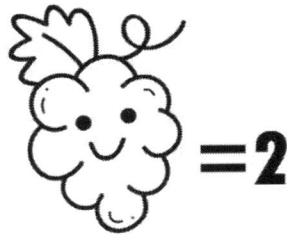

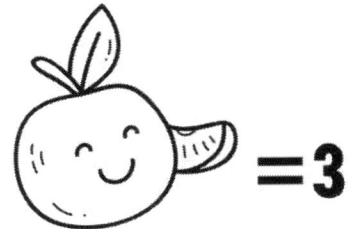

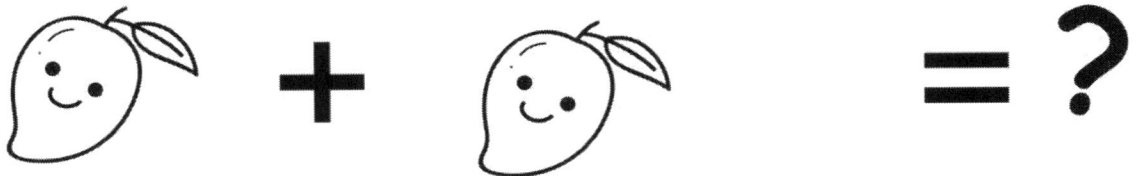

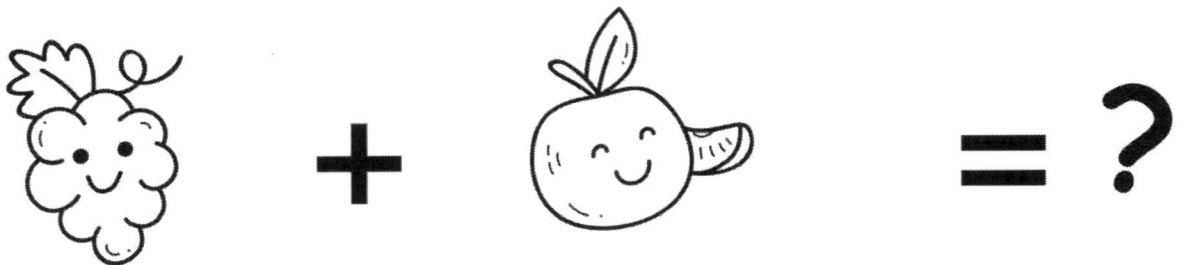

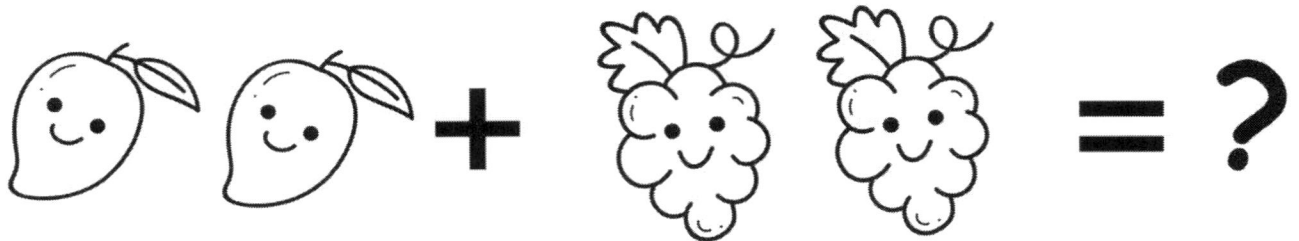

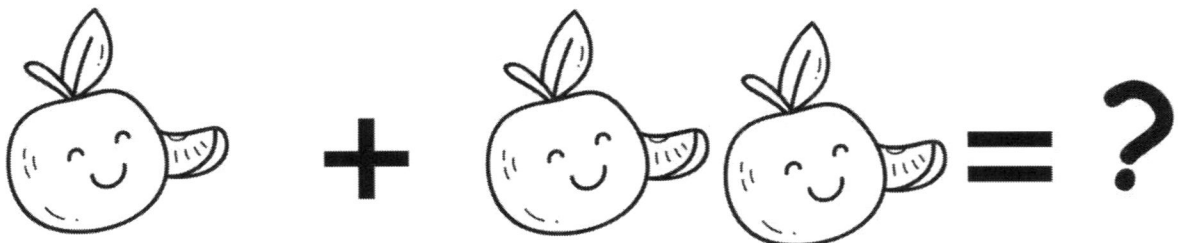

 =1   =2   =3

 + = ?

 + = ?

  +   = ?

 +   = ?

Bonus #2

Replace mango with number 1, Replace grape with number 2,
Replace apple with number 3.
What is the answer to each question?

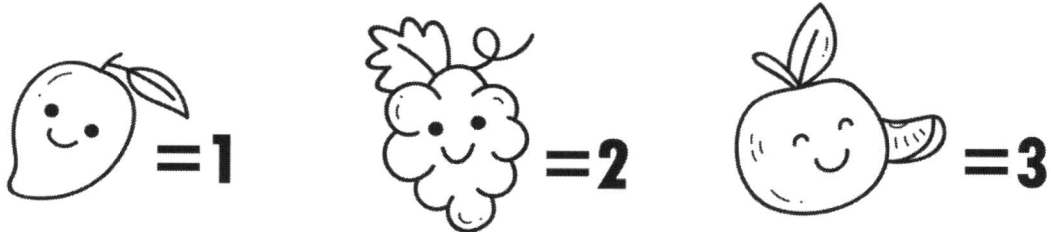

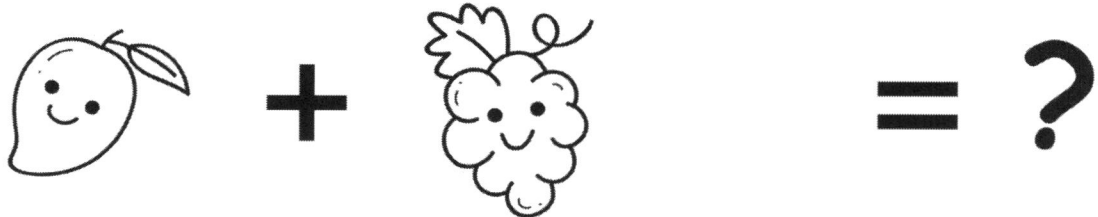

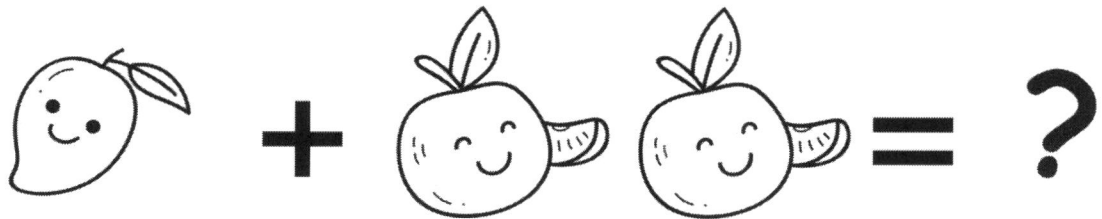

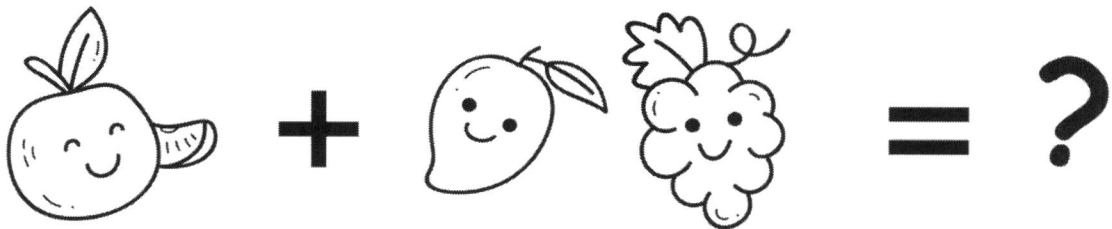

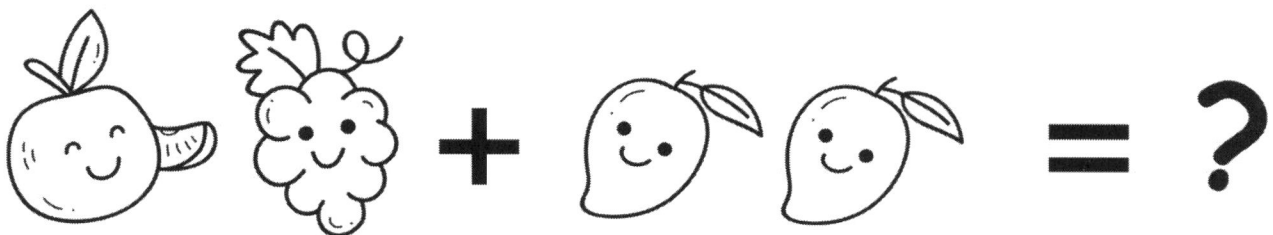

mango =1   grape =2   apple =3

mango + grape = ?

mango + apple + apple = ?

apple + mango grape = ?

apple grape + mango mango = ?

Bonus #3

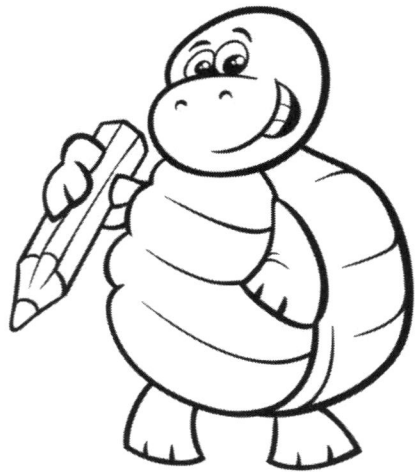

1. ② + ❓ = ⑤

2. ❓ + ③ = ⑧

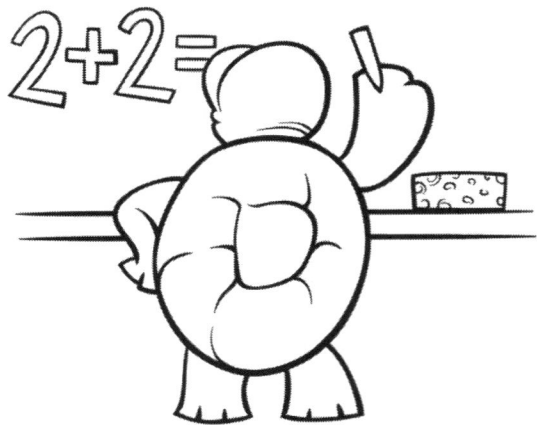

3. ❓ + ② = ④

4. ❓ + ① = ⑥

5. ⑥ + ❓ = ⑫

6. ❓ − ③ = ⑦

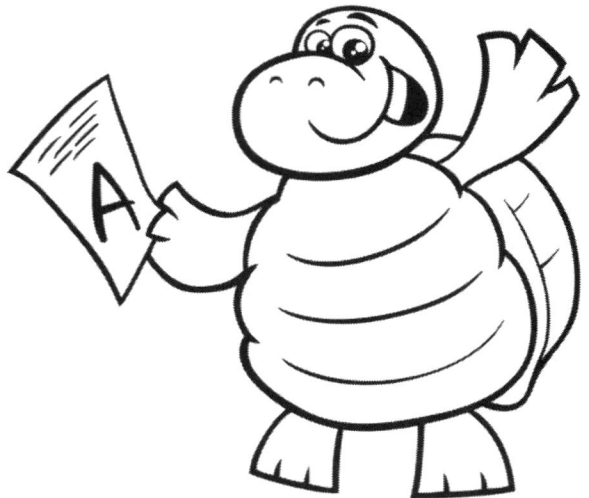

Answer 1. = _____   Answer 2. = _____   Answer 3. = _____

Answer 4. = _____   Answer 5. = _____   Answer 6. = _____

Bonus #3

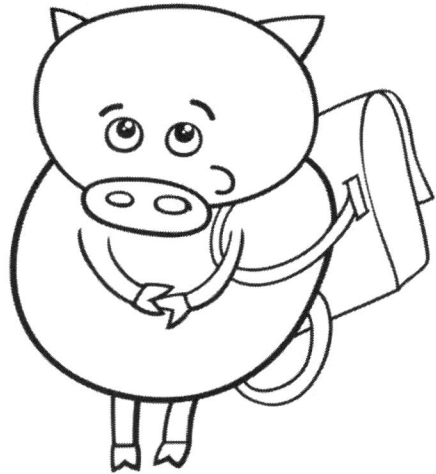

1. (?) + (6) = (7)

2. (10) – (?) = (9)

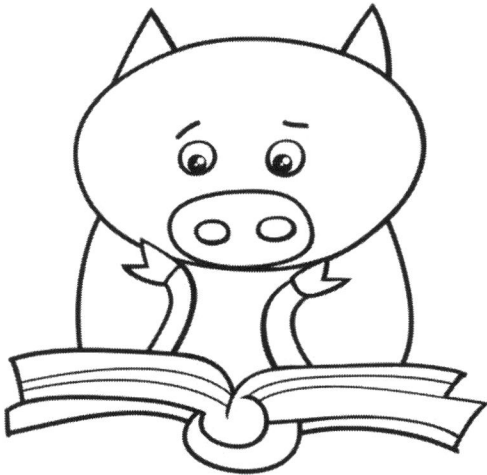

3. (4) – (?) = (2)

4. (?) + (3) = (5)

5. (?) + (4) = (14)

6. (?) (1) = (8)

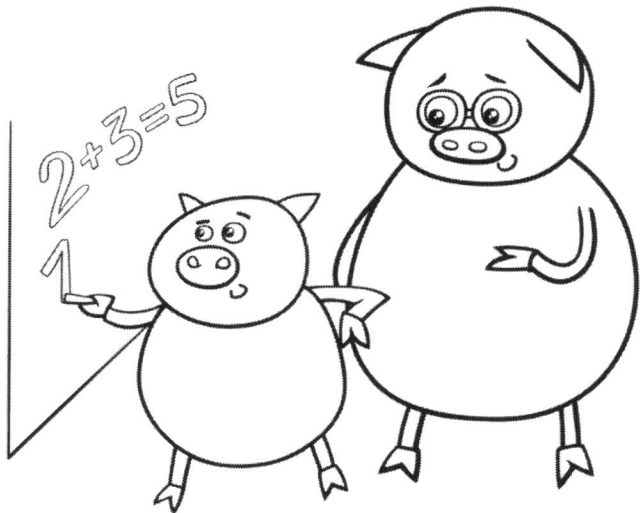

Answer 1. = _____   Answer 2. = _____   Answer 3. = _____

Answer 4. = _____   Answer 5. = _____   Answer 6. = _____

Bonus #4

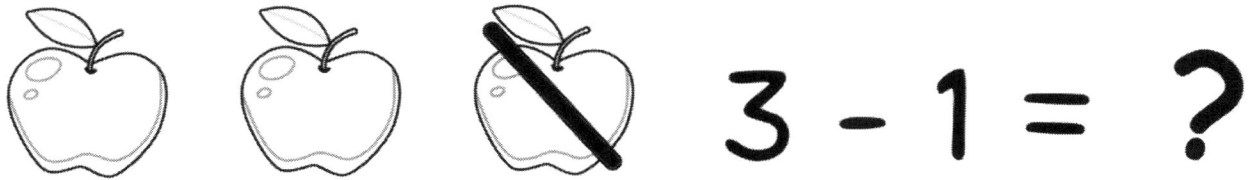 3 - 1 = ?

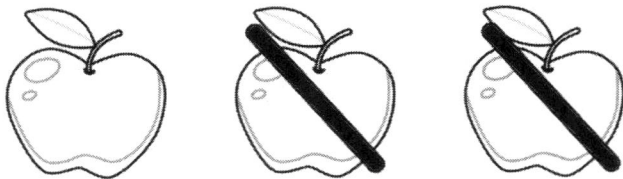 3 - 2 = ?

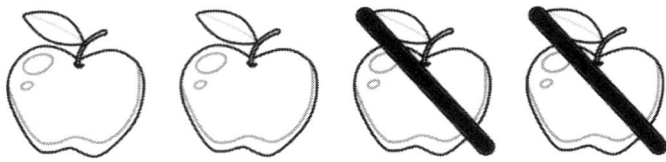 4 - 2 = ?

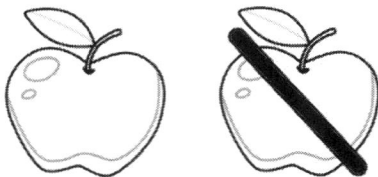 2 - 1 = ?

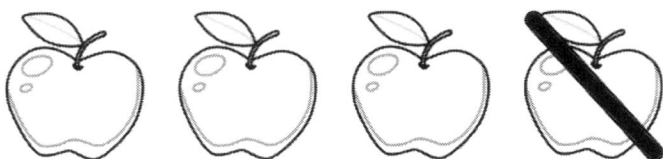 4 - 1 = ?

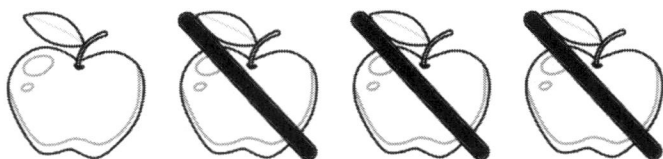 4 - 3 = ?

Bonus #4

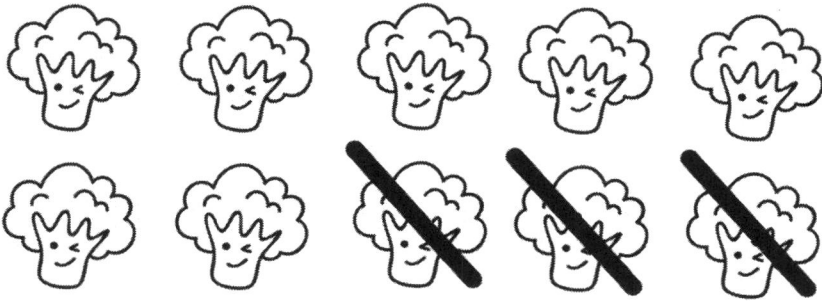

10 - 3 = ?

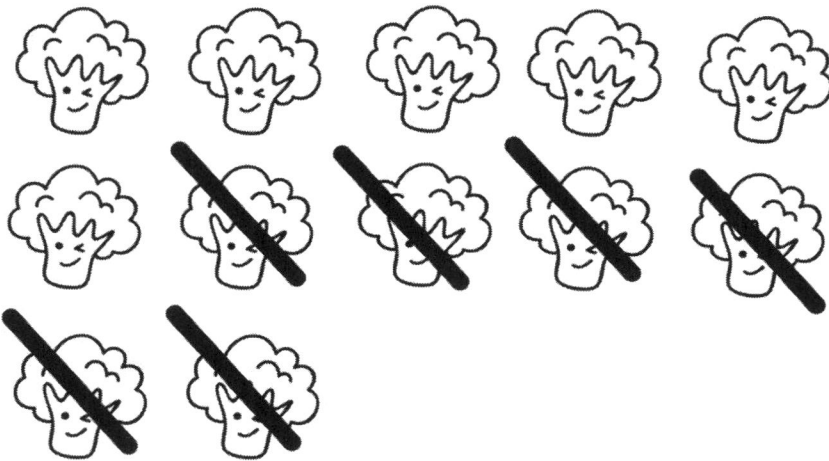

12 - 6 = ?

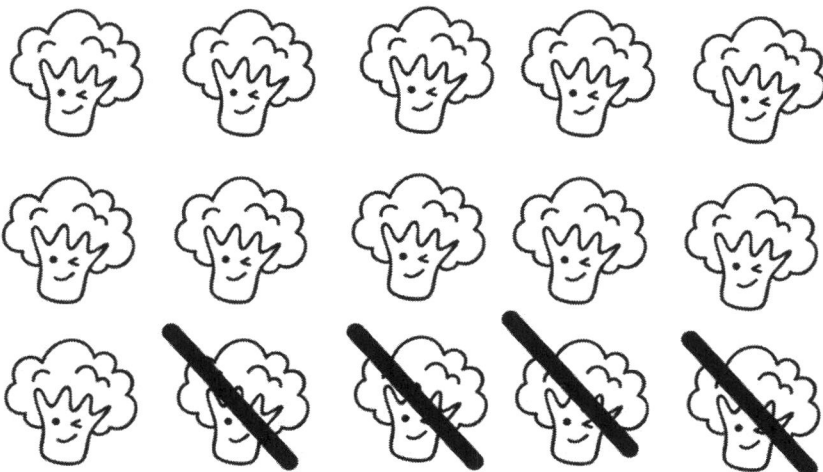

15 - 4 = ?

Answer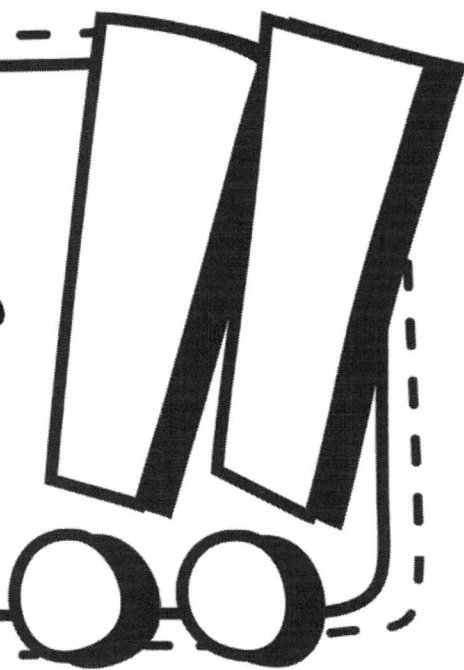

Answer Level 1

1. I am less than 10.
I am more than the number of sides on a triangle.
I am 2+2.
What number am I?
Answer : 4

2. I am more than 2.
I am less than seven.
I am one more than the toes on one foot.
What number am I?
Answer : 6

3. I am between zero and 10.
I am more than two.
I am the number before 4.
What number am I?
Answer : 3

4. I am less than 20.
I am more than the number of days in a week.
I am 7+5.
What number am I?
Answer : 12

5. I am less than 10.
I am more than three.
I am the number of sides on two squares.
What number am I?
Answer : 8

Answer Level 1

6. I am between 0 and 20.
I am more than 3+3.
I am the number of sides on two rectangles.
What number am I?
Answer : 8

7. I am between 2 and 10.
I am less than eight.
I am the number of sides on two triangles.
What number am I?
Answer : 6

8. I am less than 15.
I am more than 6+3.
I am one less than thirteen.
What number am I?
Answer : 12

9. I am between 0 and 20.
I am more than the number of sides on two rectangles.
I am 6+5.
What number am I?
Answer : 11

10. I am between 0 and 15.
I am less than 10.
I am the number of days in one week.
What number am I?
Answer : 7

Answer Level 1

11. I am between 0 and 20.
I am more than the number of fingers on two hands.
I am one less than 15.
What number am I?
Answer : 14

12. I am between 0 and 15.
I am more than 4.
I am one less than 11.
What number am I?
Answer : 10

13. I am less than 15.
I am more than 6.
I am 10 – 2.
What number am I?
Answer : 8

14. I am between 0 and 15.
I am less than nine.
I am two more than 4.
What number am I?
Answer : 6

15. I am between 0 and 20.
I am less than the number of fingers on two hands.
I am 2+5.
What number am I?
Answer : 7

Answer Level 1

16. I am between 0 and 20.
I am more than 8.
I am 7+2.
What number am I?
Answer : 9

17. I am between 0 and 20.
I am less than 15.
I am the number of sides on a triangle and a square.
What number am I?
Answer : 7

18 I am between 0 and 20.
I am more than the number of fingers on one hand.
I am 6 + 4.
What number am I?
Answer : 10

19. I am between 2 and 20.
I am more than 12.
I am 13 + 1.
What number am I?
Answer : 14

20. I am between 0 and 15.
I am less than 12.
I am 9 – 3.
What number am I?
Answer : 6

Answer Level 2

1. I am a number between 20 and 30. If you count by fives, you will say my name. Who am I?
Answer : 25

2. I am a number between 7 and 12. If you count by threes, you will say my name. Who am I?
Answer : 9

3. I am an even number. I am between 6 and 9. Who am I?
Answer : 8

4. I am a number less than 10. If you add me to myself, you will find a number greater than 16. Who am I?
Answer : 9

5. If you add me to 1, you will find an odd number. I am less than 2. Who am I?
Answer : 0

Answer Level 2

6. 16 – 10 is less than I am. 16 – 8 is greater than I am.
Who am I?
Answer : 7

7. If you subtract me from 14, you will find a
number greater than 11. I am an odd number. Who am I?
Answer : 1

8. I am an odd number. I am between 41 and 44.
Who am I?
Answer : 43

9. If you add me to 50, you will find a number less than 70.
If you count by tens you will say my name. Who am I?
Answer : 10

10. 7 + 7 is less than I am. 7 + 9 is greater than I am.
Who am I?
Answer : 15

Answer Level 3

A grandmother, two mothers, and two daughters went to a basketball game together and bought one ticket each. How many tickets did they buy in total?

Answer: 3 tickets (the grandmother is also a mother and the mother is also a daughter)

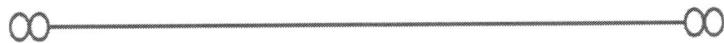

When Jackie was 6 years old, his little sister, Monica, was half is age. If Jackie is 40 years old today, how old is Monica?

Answer: She is 37 years old.

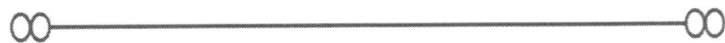

Add the number to the number itself and then multiply by 4. Again divide the number by 8 and you will get the same number once more. Which is that number?

Answer: Any number

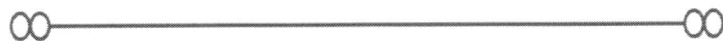

I add five to nine, and get two. The answer is correct, but how?

Answer: When it is 9am, add 5 hours to it and you will get 2pm.

Answer Level 3

Eggs are $0.12 a dozen. How many eggs can you get for a dollar?

Answer: 100 eggs, at one penny each

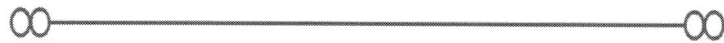

∞———————————————————∞

A man is twice as old as his little sister. He is also half as old as their dad. Over a period of 50 years, the age of the sister will become half of their dad's age. What is the age of the man now?

Answer: He is 50 years old.

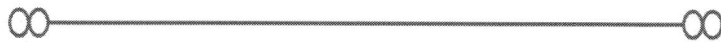

∞———————————————————∞

The ages of a father and son add up to 66. The father's age is the son's age reversed. How old could they be?

Answer: There are three possible solutions for this, the father-son duo could be 51 and 15 years old, 42 and 24 years old or 60 and 06 years old.

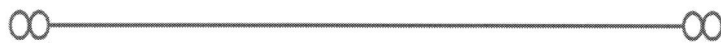

∞———————————————————∞

There are 100 pairs of bears in a zoo. Two pairs of babies are born for every dog. Unfortunately, 23 of the bears have not survived. How many bears would be left in total?

Answer: 977 bears
(100 x 2 = 200; 200 + 800 = 1000; 1000 – 23 = 977)

Answer Level 3

Charlie has two kids. If the elder kid is a boy, then what is the possibility that his other kid is also a boy?

Answer: 50 percent

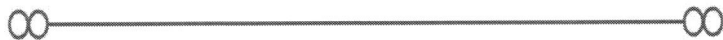

∞———————————∞

Velma has 7 daughters and each of them has a brother. Can you figure out the total number of kids Velma have?

Answer: 8 kids because the sisters have just one brother in common.

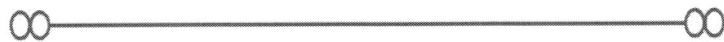

∞———————————∞

A little boy goes shopping and purchases 12 potatoes. On the way home, all but 9 get mushed and ruined. How many potatoes are left in a good condition?

Answer: 9

∞———————————∞

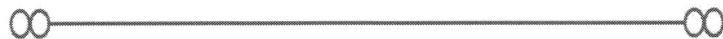

If you had five oranges and two apples in one hand and two oranges and four apples in the other hand, what would you have?

Answer: Very Large Hands

Answer Level 4

1. Kevin turned 10 years old day before yesterday.
By next year he will become 13. How is this possible?

Answer: we need to assume that today is 1st January 2019.
This means that Kevin's eleventh birthday was
on 31st December 2018.
Day before yesterday, he was 10 years old,
today he is 11. By the end of the current year, 2019,
he will be 12 years old. And so, by the next year (i.e. in 2020),
he will be 13 years old.

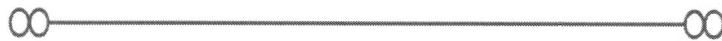

∞────────────────────────────∞

2. What is the following number?
18, 21, 24, 27, 30, 33, 36, _____

Answer: Every successive number is greater by 3.
So the sequence will be:
18, 21, 24, 27, 30, 33, 36, 39, 42, 45, 48, and so on.

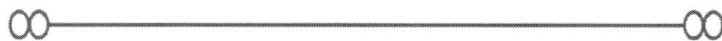

∞────────────────────────────∞

3. What is the following number?
53, 51, 49, 47, 45, 43, _____

Answer: Every successive number is smaller by 2.
So the sequence will be:
53, 51, 49, 47, 45, 43, 41, 39, 37, 35, and so on.

Answer Level 4

4. David had 6 siblings who were born all born 2 years apart. The youngest is Lila who is only 7 years old while David is the oldest. What is David's age?

Answer: Lila, the youngest sibling is 7 years old. Each sibling was born 2 years apart, and there are total seven children (David and his 6 siblings). So David's age is: 7 + 2 + 2 + 2 + 2 + 2 + 2 = 19.

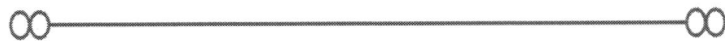

5. Two fathers and two sons go fishing. Each of them catches one fish. So why do they bring home only three fish?

Answer: The fishing group comprises a grandfather, his son, and his son's son. So, there are just three people.

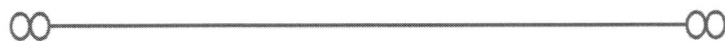

6. If Ella is the 50th fastest and slowest runner in her school, how many students are there in her school?

Answer: 99 students.

50th Fastest Calculation:
If you count in sequence from 1, Ella comes 50.
50th Slowest Calculation:
If you count in sequence from 99, Ella is again 50.

Answer Level 4

7. Wolves and Lambs Puzzles: Six Wolves can catch just six lambs in six minutes. So how many wolves will they need to catch 60 lambs in sixty minutes?
Hint – the answer is not sixty.

Answer: 1 wolf can catch 1 lamb in six minutes.
In 60 minutes, each wolf can catch 10 lambs.
So, each wolf can catch ten lambs, and in sixty minutes, 6 wolves can catch 60 lambs. Another method – Six Wolves.
How? 6 wolves can catch six lambs in 6 minutes.
If you multiply it by ten, the same wolves can catch sixty lambs in 60 minutes.

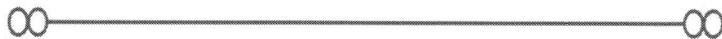

8. What do the numbers 88, 96 and 11 all have in common?

Answer: They look the same upside down and right side up.

Answer Level 4

9. There are 2 buckets, a 5 litre and a 3-litre bucket.
Fill the 5-litre bucket with 4 litres of water using just
these two buckets to measure.

Answer: Fill the 5-litre bucket fully. Pour it into
the 3-litre bucket until it is full. Empty the 3-litre bucket.
Pour the remaining 2 litres into the 3-litre bucket.
Fill the 5-litre bucket completely. Finish filling
the 3-litre bucket. Now the 5-litre bucket is left
with exactly 4 litres of water.

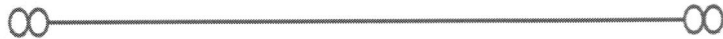

10. rabbit and carrots: Another word problem that is fun
for kids to solve. Assume there are, five rabbits
and each one takes 5 minutes to eat 5 carrots.
How many minutes would 4 rabbits take to eat 4 carrots?
Again, how many rabbits would eat 30 carrots in 30 minutes?

Answer: Each rabbit eats 5 carrots in 5 minutes,
so 1 carrot in 1 minute. So, if there are 4 rabbits
and 4 carrots, they will take 1 minute only.
On the other hand, if 30 carrots are being
eaten in 30 minutes (i.e. 1 carrot in 1 minute),
this is the job of one rabbit.

Answer Level 4

11. What weighs more – A kilo of apples or a kilo of feathers?

Answer: They weigh the same. Each weighs exactly a kilo.

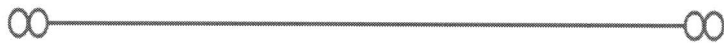

∞————————————————∞

12. Using only addition, how can you add eight 8's to get the number 1,000?

Answer: 888 + 88 + 8 + 8 + 8 =1,000

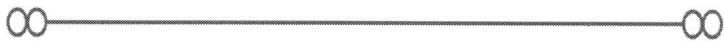

∞————————————————∞

13. The ages of a father and son add up to 66. The age of the dad is the age of the son reversed. How old could they be?

Answer: There are three different answers for this: the father and son could be 51 and 15 years or 42 and 24 years old or 60 and 06 years old.

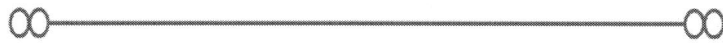

∞————————————————∞

14. How many 9's are there between 1 and 100?

Answer: 20.
They are 9,19,29,39,49,59,69,79,89,90,91,92,93,94,95, 96,97,98,99

Answer Level 5

1. When Grant was 8, his brother was half his age. Now, Grant is 14. How old is his brother?

Answer :
His brother is 10.
Half of 8 is 4, so Grant's brother is 4 years younger.
This means when Grant is 14, his brother is
still 4 years younger, so he's 10.

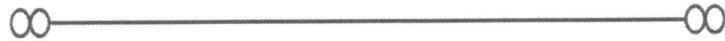

2. Two fathers and 2 sons spent the day fishing, but only caught 3 fish. This was enough for each of them to have one fish. How is this possible?

Answer :
There were only 3 people fishing.
There was one father, his son, and his son's son.
This means there were 2 fathers and 2 sons,
since one of them is a father and a son.

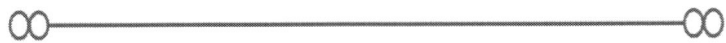

3. Leo was 11 the day before yesterday, and next year he'll turn 14. How is this possible?

Answer :
Today is January 1st, and Leo's birthday is December 31st.
Leo was 11 the day before yesterday (December 30th),
then turned 12 the next day. This year on December 31st
he'll turn 13, so next year he'll turn 14.

Answer Level 5

4. Isabella has 5 daughters. Each of these daughters has a brother. How many children does Isabella have?

Answer :
She has 6 children.
Each daughter has the same brother.
There are 5 daughters and 1 son.

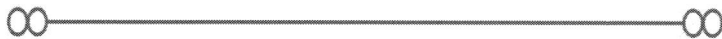

5. It's raining at midnight, but the forecast for tomorrow and the next day is clear. Will there be sunny weather in 48 hours?

Answer :
No, it won't be sunny because it will be dark out.
In 48 hours, it will be midnight again.

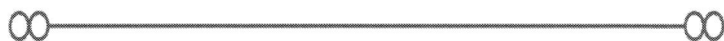

6. There are 3 apples in the basket and you take away 2. How many apples do you have now?

Answer :
You have 2 apples.
You took away 2 apples and left 1 in the basket.

Answer Level 5

7. What can you put between 7 and 8, to make the result greater than 7, but less than 8?

Answer :
A decimal point.
Your result would be 7.8, which is between 7 and 8.

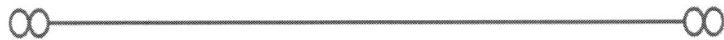

8. What 3 numbers give the same result when multiplied and added together?

Answer :
1, 2, and 3.
1 + 2 + 3 = 6
1 x 2 x 3 = 6

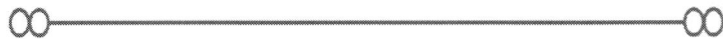

9. 81 x 9 = 801. What do you need to do to make this equation true?

Answer :
Turn it upside down.
108 = 6 x 18.

Answer Level 6

1. This means that if the genie came on the 20th,
he would need 20 grams of gold. What did Charlie do next?

Answer: This is a challenging math riddle for kids as
the date is unknown. If Charlie decided to make a different
gold ring for each day, it will become problematic.
This is because he only has a 100 grams of gold. So,
if he made a gold ring of 31 grams,30 grams, 29 grams
and 27 grams, he would run out of gold. The solution is to
make just 5 rings of weight 1 gram, 2 grams, 4 grams,
8 grams and 16 grams. This can be used in combination
to reach the number 31.

For example:

24th day: 16+8
13th day: 8+4+1
7th day: 4+2+1

Answer Level 6

2. How Many Cycles? This is another mathematical statement problem which can be solved using logic and arithmetic. Last weekend, Jack went to play in the park near his house. He rode the new bicycle gifted by his grandma on his birthday. After reaching the park, Jack saw that there were 14 tricycles and bicycles. If there were totally 38 wheels, how many tricycles were there in the park?

Answer: There were 10 Tricycles.
There were 14 cycles in all, and all of them have at least 2 wheels. So, 14 x 2 = 28. Now there are 38 wheels totally, which means 38 – 28 = 10. So, this means there are 10 cycles with one extra wheel each, meaning 10 tricycles in all.

Answer Level 6

3. Three brothers live in a farm. They agreed to buy new seeds: James and Thomas would go and Charlie stayed to protect fields. Thomas bought 75 sacks of wheat in the market whereas James bought 45 sacks. At home, they split the sacks equally. Charlie had paid 1400 dollars for the wheat. How much dollars did Thomas and James get of the sum, considering equal split of the sacks?

Answer: Thomas $1225, James $175

Every farmer's part is 1/3(45+75)=40 sacks.
Charlie paid $1400 for 40 sacks,
then 1 sack costs $1400/40=$35/sack.

James got $35 x (45-40)=35 x 5=$175.
Thomas got $35 x (75-40)=35 x 35=$1225.

Answer Level 6

4. In reply to an inquiry about the animals on his farm, the farmer says: "I only ever keep sheep, pigs, and horses. In fact, at the moment they are all sheep bar three, all pigs bar four, and all horses bar five." How many does he have of each animal?

Answer: The farmer has 3 sheep, 2 pigs, 1 horse. Adding 3, 4, and 5, in this case, gives twice the number of animals, so there must be six animals altogether.

Answer Bonus #1

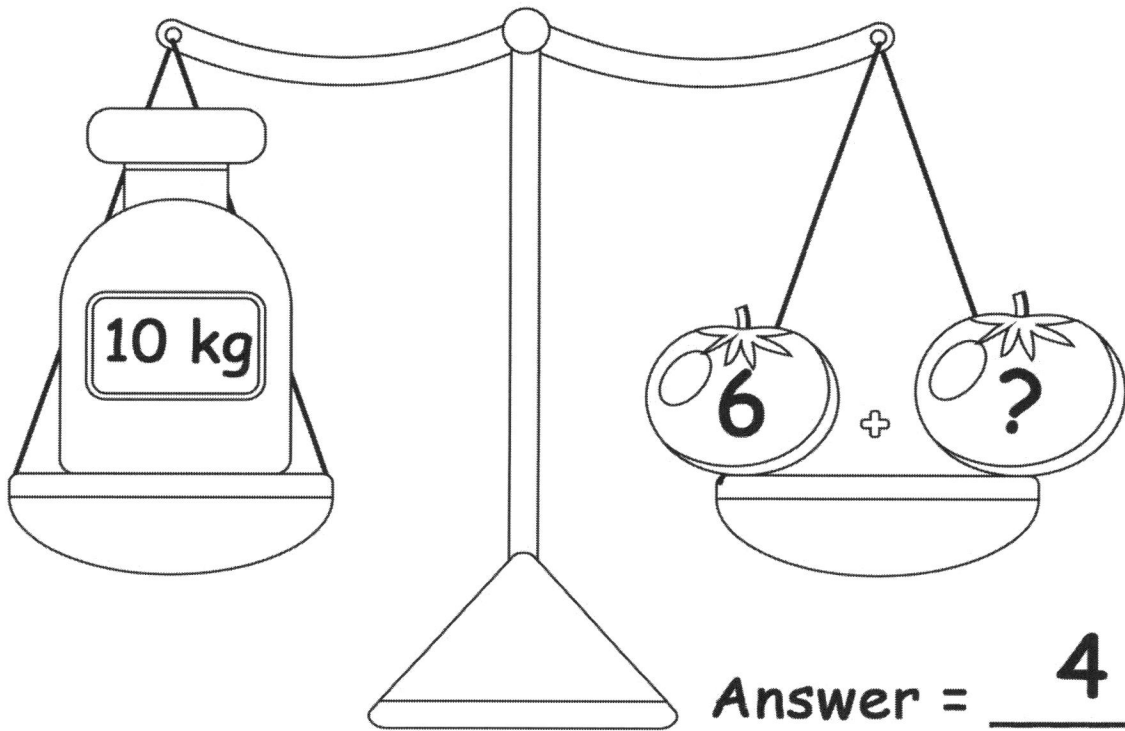

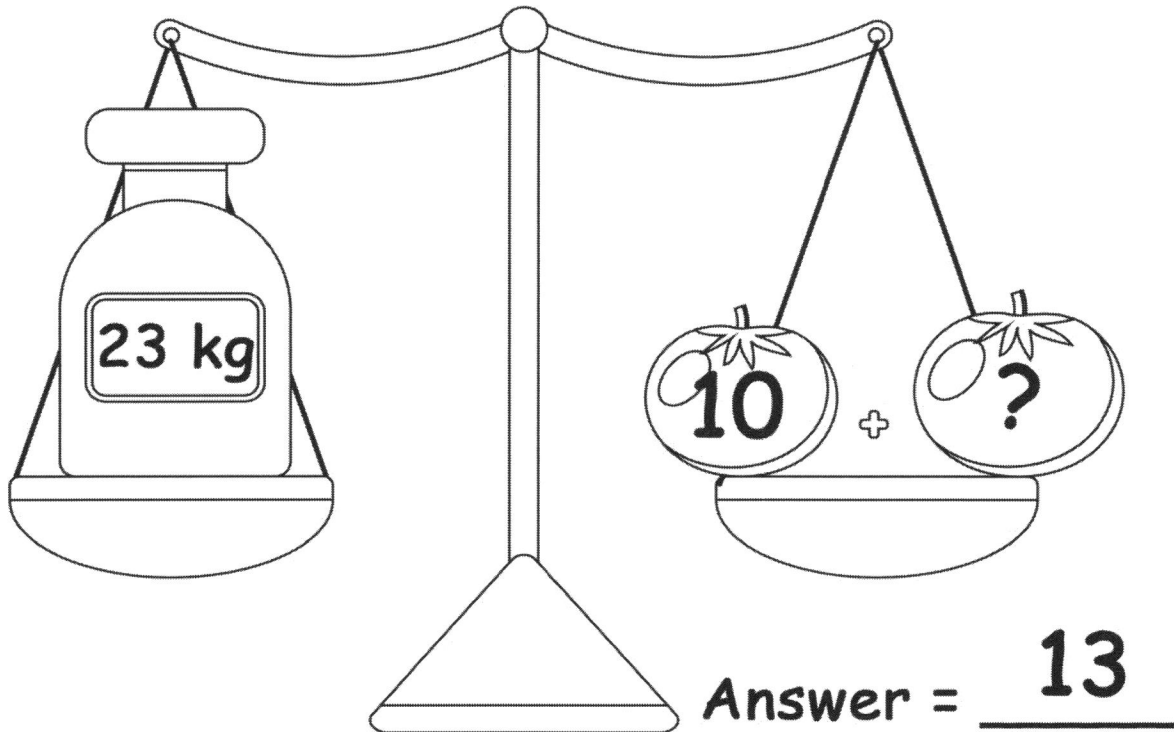

10 kg

6 + ?

Answer = ___4___

23 kg

10 + ?

Answer = ___13___

Answer Bonus #1

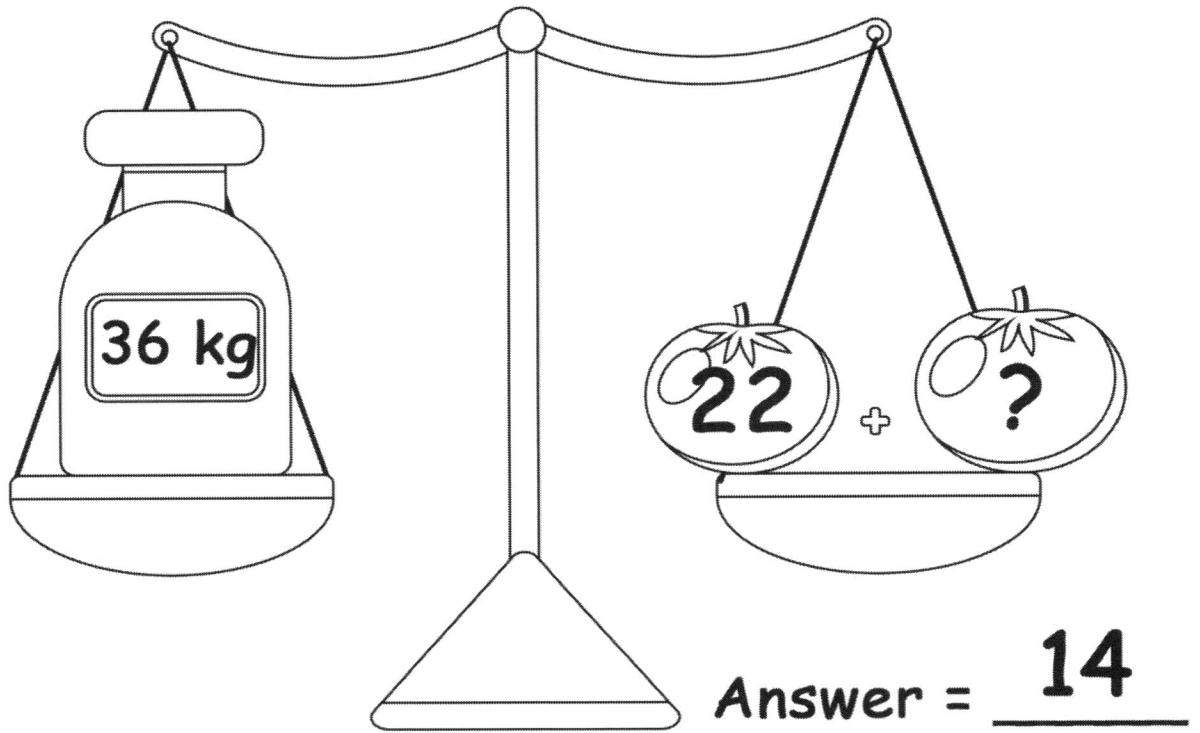

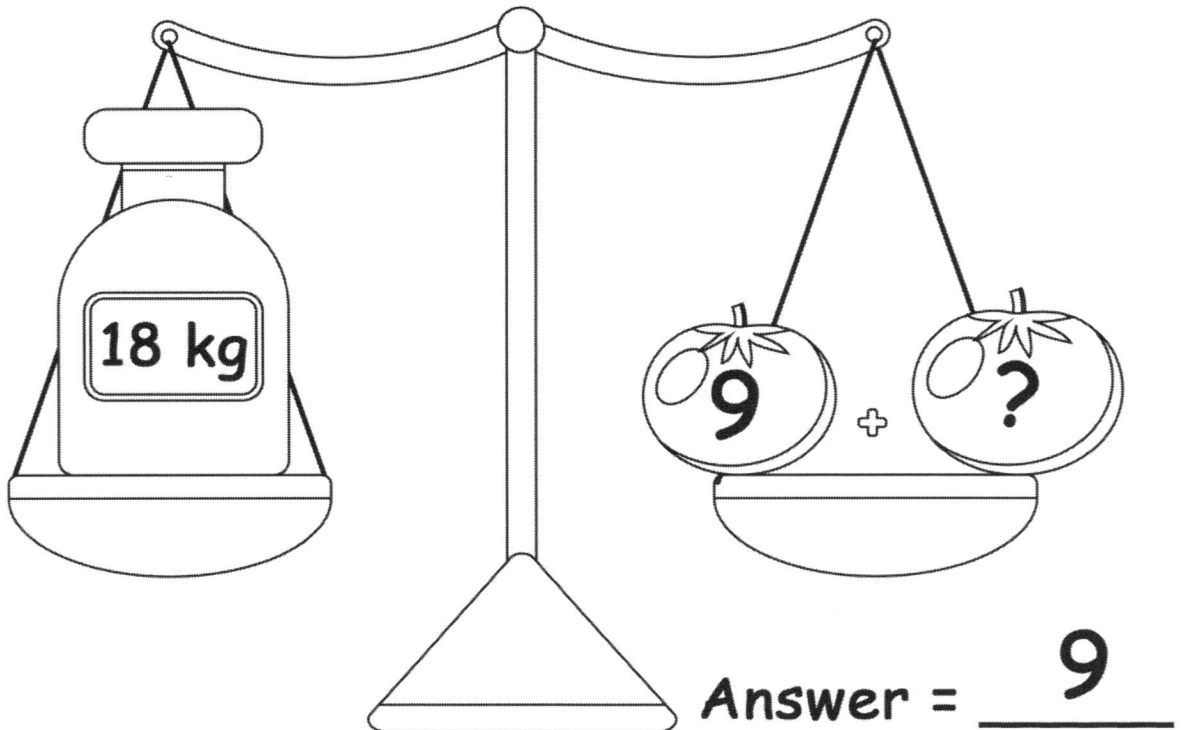

36 kg

22 + ?

Answer = 14

18 kg

9 + ?

Answer = 9

Answer Bonus #2

Replace mango with number 1, Replace grape with number 2,
Replace apple with number 3.
What is the answer to each question?

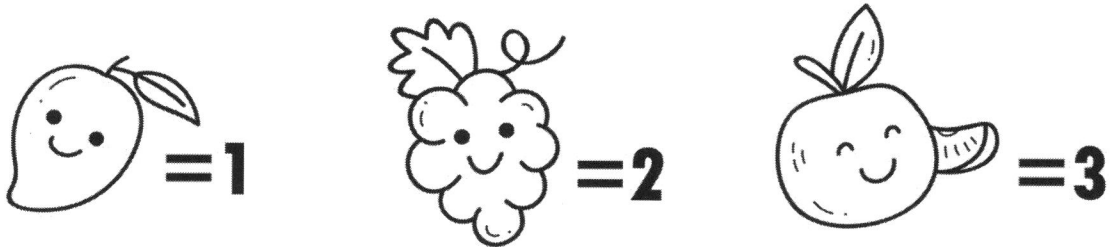

mango =1   grape =2   apple =3

mango (1) + mango (1) = 2

grape (2) + apple (3) = 5

mango mango (11) + grape grape (22) = 33

apple (3) + apple apple (33) = 36

Answer Bonus #2

Replace mango with number 1, Replace grape with number 2,
Replace apple with number 3.
What is the answer to each question?

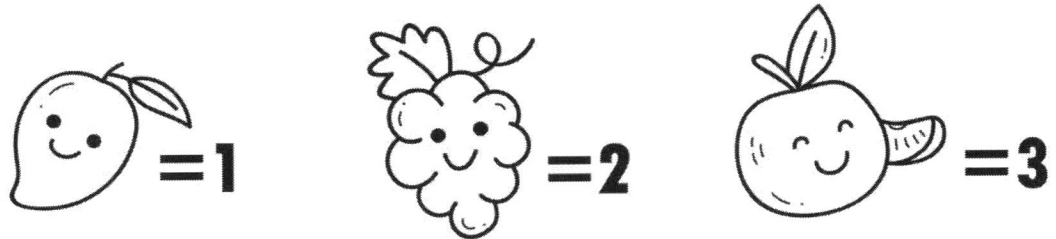

🥭 =1   🍇 =2   🍎 =3

🥭 + 🍇 = 3
(1)   (2)

🥭 + 🍎🍎 = 34
(1)   (33)

🍎 + 🥭🍇 = 15
(3)   (12)

🍎🍇 + 🥭🥭 = 43
(32)   (11)

Answer Bonus #3

1. ② + ? = ⑤

2. ? + ③ = ⑧

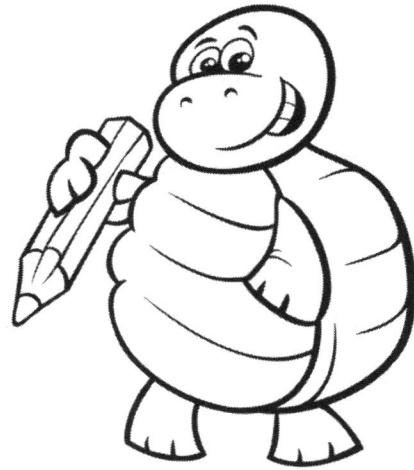

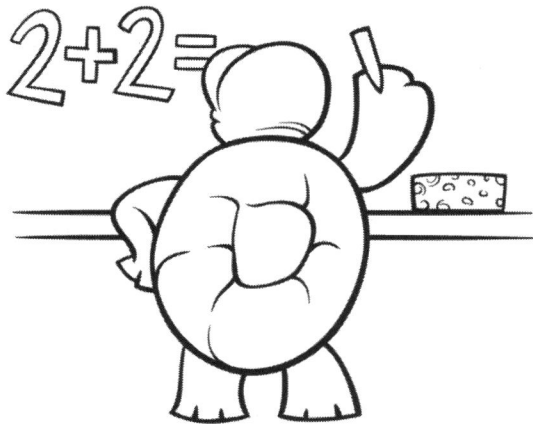

3. ? + ② = ④

4. ? + ① = ⑥

5. ⑥ + ? = ⑫

6. ? − ③ = ⑦

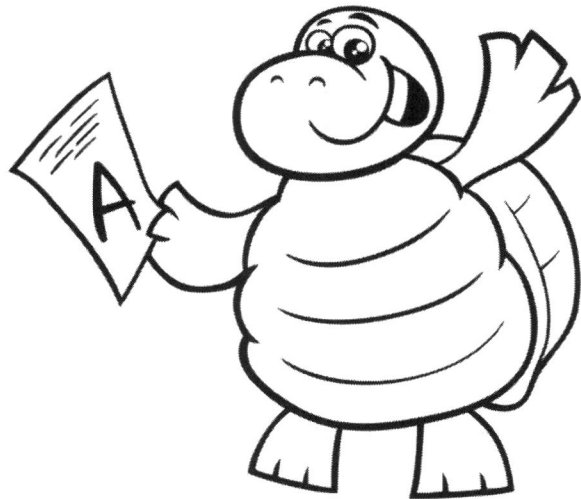

Answer 1. = __3__   Answer 2. = __5__   Answer 3. = __2__

Answer 4. = __5__   Answer 5. = __6__   Answer 6. = __10__

Answer Bonus #3

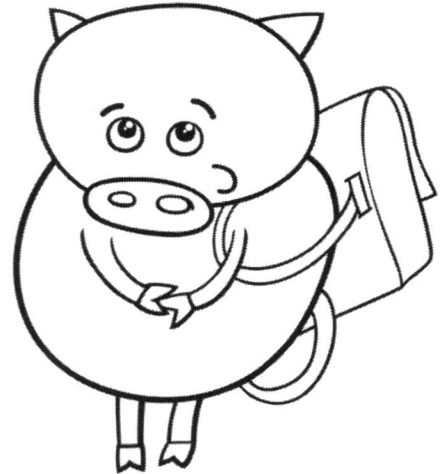

1. (?) + (6) = (7)

2. (10) − (?) = (9)

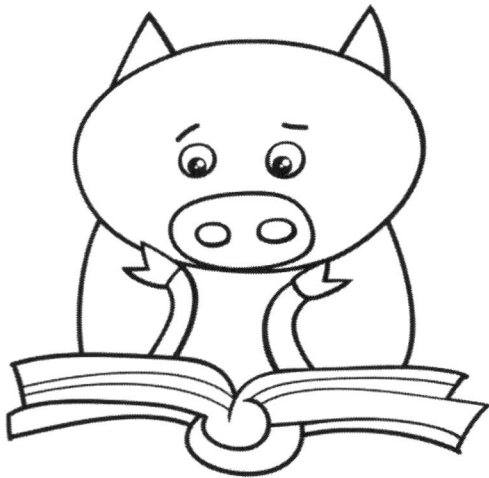

3. (4) − (?) = (2)

4. (?) + (3) = (5)

5. (?) + (4) = (14)

6. (?) − (1) = (8)

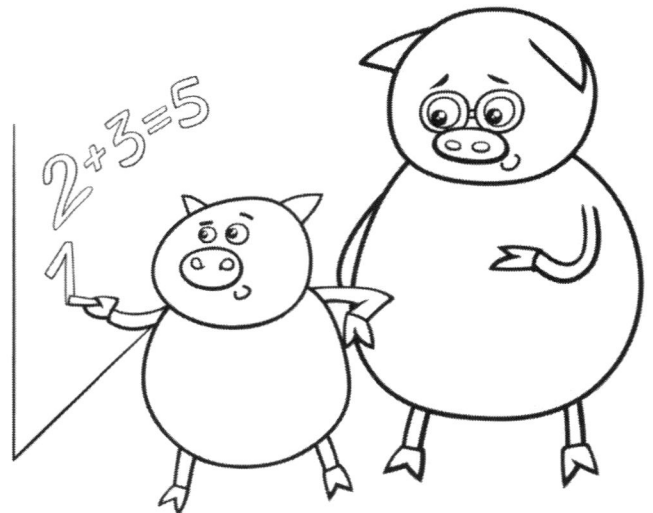

Answer 1. = __1__   Answer 2. = __1__   Answer 3. = __2__

Answer 4. = __2__   Answer 5. = __10__   Answer 6. = __9__

Answer Bonus #4

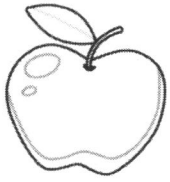 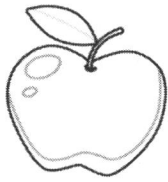 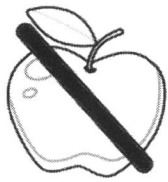 3 - 1 = 2

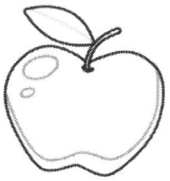 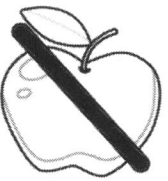 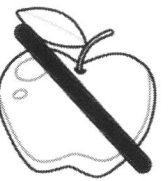 3 - 2 = 1

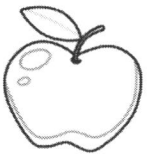 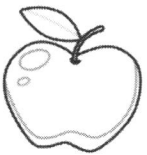 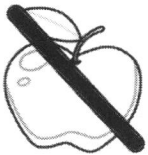 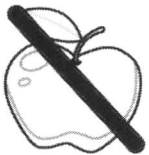 4 - 2 = 2

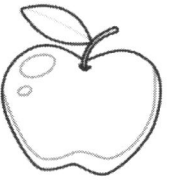 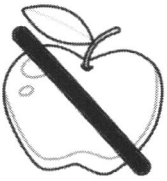 2 - 1 = 1

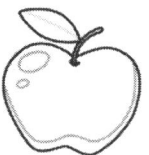 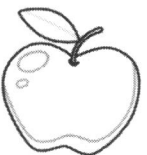 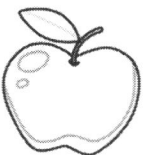 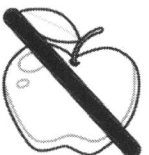 4 - 1 = 3

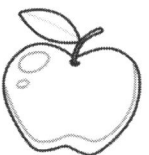 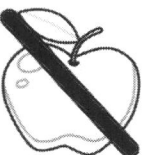 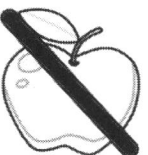 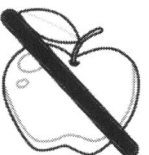 4 - 3 = 1

Answer Bonus #4

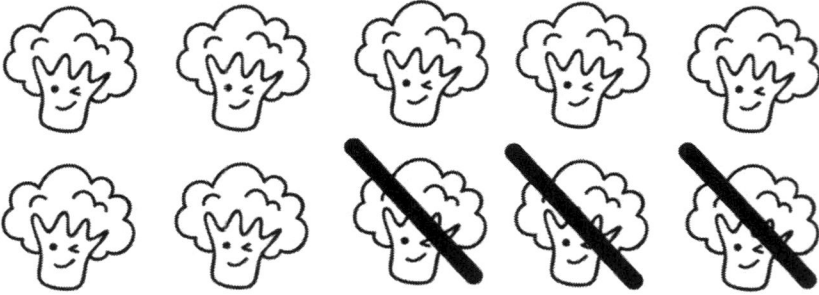

$$10 - 3 = 7$$

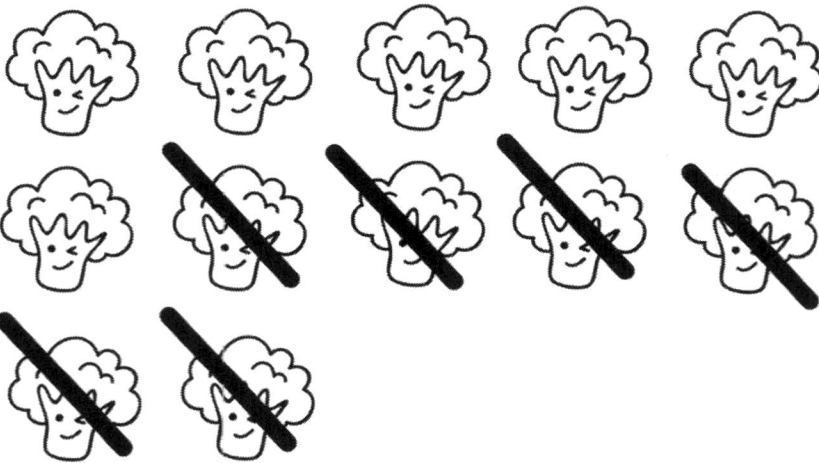

$$12 - 6 = 6$$

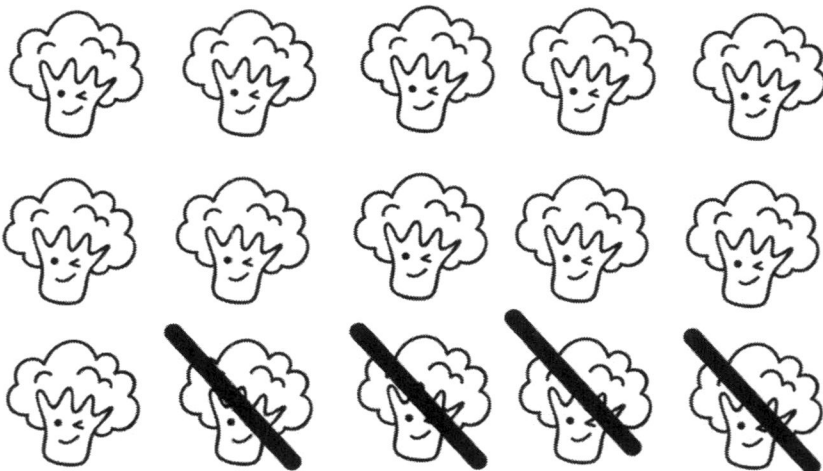

$$15 - 4 = 11$$

Printed in Great Britain
by Amazon